MW01268828

SEX POSITIONS

FOR COUPLES

SECRETS

AN EASY-TO-FOLLOW GUIDE TO THE
BEST SEX POSITIONS EVERY COUPLE
SHOULD TRY IN ORDER TO BOOST
YOUR COUPLE'S PLEASURE AND
IMPROVE INTIMACY IN YOUR
RELATIONSHIP

ALICIA GREY

© Copyright 2021 - All rights reserved.

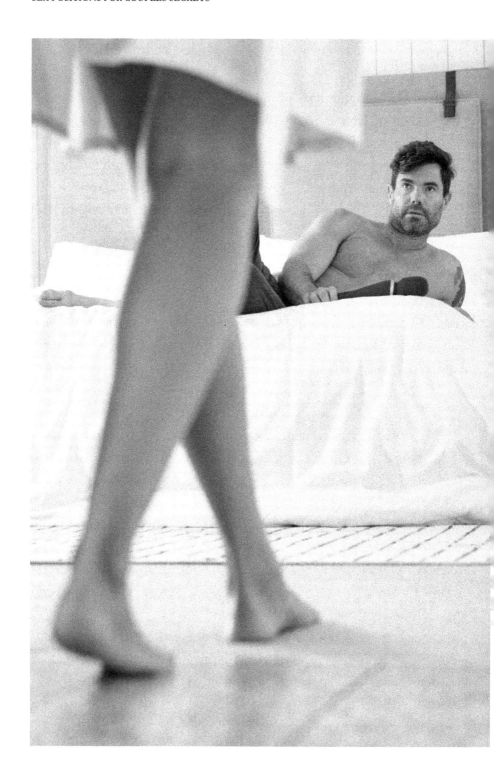

Table of Contents

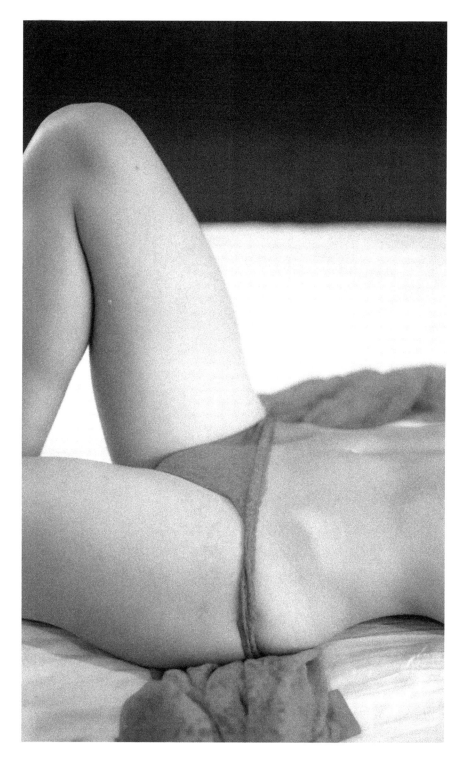

Introduction

So, what is BDSM? You may be asking yourself this question after reading 50 Shades or seeing 50 Shades freed in theaters. You begin to wonder if it is anything like what Christian Grey did to Anna. The truth is, it is not, and this form does teeter way closer to the level of abuse. But what exactly is it? Why is it something that is considered "pleasurable" for another person? After all, I may seem like something that you should not do, since it does involve hurting another person. Why hurt someone? Why relinquish control? Well, read on, and we will discuss what it is, and why it matters.

BDSM by definition, in the most basic, unadulterated form, is bondage and discipline/dominance and submission or sado-masochism. What that means is that it is an umbrella term that has underneath it any sexual act or mindset that involves two things and they are:

- Dominating

- Relinquishing control

Now, it might seem weird that BDSM is just that after all, why would people relinquish control in the bedroom? The answer is that it can be super liberating, and in the long run, if you engage in it, will turn you on in quite a different way compared to other forms of sex.

You've probably looked up BDSM, and you've seen those girls strapped to something tight. You cringe maybe at the guy smacking her, since you can hear the sounds echoing the truth as well is, that BDSM is a very umbrella term, meaning that yes, it involves that. Still, it also involves having your partner refer to you as sir or madam. It can be a wide variety of things, and it is something that you have to realize, is something that has different standards.

You might see the media representation of this as something silly and seedy, or taboo in a sense. However, with new liberation in sexual freedom, the rise of women wanting to take more control of their bodies, and the exploration of sexuality, this type of sexual endeavor is something that many have started to come in contact with, and one that's interested many.

Why This Play is good

This play can change the mental state of your body, in different types of ways.

That is because, when you are doing this, you are releasing endorphins in the body. Every time you are in pain, or there is some type of experience is occurring, your body will release these "happy hormones" and you will feel really good.

This can be extremely liberating for both the Dom and the sub since it can release these feelings in both of their minds.

Now, when you are doing this, you should always make sure that you both are cool with exploring them. But, when you do relinquish this type of control, allow for your partner to do the bidding, this creates trust.

Trust is something that many people struggle with sometimes. They feel like they always have to be on guard, or in control. But sometimes not being in control is pretty great. Allowing another person to take control consensually and safely can be an amazing feeling. There is not anything "wrong" with that. Being pampered and taken care of in different ways, allowing your body to feel different sensations, and overall pleasure in this form can be quite liberating, and extremely stimulating.

If you have never done this before, it is always worth a try. It can be quite different, but it is pretty nice.

You are both on Equal Ground

The biggest thing that you must remember when you are doing this is that you are both on equal ground when it comes to this, and the distribution of power. When you are doing this with your domestic partner, you also want to be on equal ground, but if you are searching out a Dom, or wanting to try this, you should keep this in mind.

In essence, this means that the power is equal between you both when you are discussing various things.

Now, this does not mean that in the scene you have equal power. That would mean that you are not experiencing BDDM. BDSM involves relinquishing some control in the form of a Dom and a sub. Still, when you are negotiating, you always, ALWAYS, need to make sure that you are both on equal playing feelings.

This is important because it will address the wants and the needs that not only you have, but what the other persons wants and needs as well. This is very important for both parties, because if you are both not on equal footing, this is how upsets and problems happen.

When you are negotiating this type of contract in the submissive role, you might run the risk of relinquishing your power and consenting to things that you usually would not consent to.

But, if you are doing this with a partner, you both sit down and talk it out. Discuss what you want and need, discuss the aftercare procedures, and discuss anything that you feel is important to your personal needs. This goes for doms, subs, and switches too. Seriously, talk this out before you get yourself into a situation you do not want to be in.

Opt in

When you are putting together a BDSM relationship, whether it be both you and your partner, or an actual contract, opting in is a crucial thing. In essence, when you "opt in" to something, it is what you are saying yes to.

In essence, it's what you want, and what you don't want when you're putting together a BDSM contract, you always want to add in the opt in parts that you're into, rather than just the opt out method.

Lots of times, we only focus on the opt out parts of relationships, which are essentially the off-limits part of this, and the deal breaker. If you do this, you will say no to things you do not want, but you might also not say what you do want, and that can then make things a little blurrier.

When you are only thinking of what you do not want to do, it can make the whole relationship a lot more confusing and create way more misunderstandings.

Chapter 1

Advanced Role-Playing Games

How often do you engage in role-playing and what is your opinion about it? We personally believe that sex games and role play are an excellent way to improve the kind of sex life you are having simply because it creates a different kind of passion.

So, if you want to do something kinky and maybe experiment with games and role play, we totally recommend you to be up for it. There are several kinds of challenges that you can throw at each other as this tends to rev up the excitement among the couples and gives them something new to hold on and explore as well.

So, let us talk of some of the possible sex games and then move on to the kind of role pay antics you could engage in.

The Striped Down Twister

We have all heard and played the classic board game twister. You have to play it the same way, the only difference is that every time someone fails, they have to remove a layer of clothing until someone strips completely and you can then move to the bed and take the game to a different level altogether.

Truth or Dare

Give the classic truth or dare a strip twist. The questions should all be related to sex or the sexual fantasy you have and the ones you have lived. When it comes to daring, have sex-related dares, it could be things like give me a blow job, strip for me, give me a lap dance, and do pole dance or anything else. The only thing you need to remember here is that the game should be played with mutual consent and the boundaries should be well decided beforehand.

The Sex Dice

You could buy the sex dice from an adult store or you could make two sets of notes yourself. In one of them, you should jot down the name of the body parts and in the other one; it should be the sexual actions that you have to do.

One partner will take out the note from one set and the other from the next one. All you have to do is perform the action on the selected body part and thereby see who what bests. This is a great way to have fun in bed.

Of course, there are endless more games. Any board game can be turned into a sex game by giving it a strip angle. Every time you lose, you will have to remove one pair of clothing. Even challenge games could be turned to sex games by giving a sex-related dare at the end of the round.

So, make full use of your imagination and let sex be the torchbearer to the games to give you a fun-filled night.

The Role-Play Sessions
Why should you do it?

When we are talking of role-play sessions, the very first thing which we are going to talk about is why you should at all engage in it. We have some clear reasons for you to do so.

☐ Sets the momentum for the rest of the sexy night to follow

☐ It is a great way to spice things up

☐ Makes you feel different

☐ Helps partners come closer and are experimental

☐ Great way to keep sex fun

☐ Offers plenty of room to try new things

So, now that the reasons are clear, we are now going to focus on some of the possible role play ideas which will give you the incentive to try them tonight with your partner. Remember, the sky is the limit when it comes to these games and once you get a hang of it; you would have a hard time letting it go.

The Professor and Student
Who does not love a good college romance? We have all fantasized about one or the other of our teachers in schools and colleges where our hormones had always been on a rage.

So, one of you could be a professor and make sure to wear a tie and glasses and strip the rest. This makes you a very sexy professor; indeed, you could use a ruler in hand or even chalk to go with the image.

When the other one is dressed like a college girl, go for pigtails or even braided hair. You could wear red lipstick and wear a sexy school uniform.

The Boss and Employee

Once you are done with the college romance, why not head to the office room right away? Your man could be a mean boss and he could wear a coat and let go of the pants. The man needs to have a stern and strict voice.

The woman could dress like a regular employee or better she could just be wearing the heels and then for the scene, you could narrate things like, "Oops, I forgot my attire, will you let me off the hook, boss?"

The idea here is to have a desk and make each other horny. Try and hint at hot, angry sex and the employee could be submissive and the boss could play the dominant role.

The Doctor and Nurse

Who said hospitals cannot be fun! You could play the role of a naughty, slutty nurse, and a sleazy doctor whose hands end up slipping on the nurse's butt every time he wants to operate.

The scene can get downright sexy and you have the option to play it anyways. The nurse could complain about possible pain in her vagina and the doctor could finger her to see what is amiss.

Once again, it all comes down to your imagination and one thing is for sure, there is no denying the fact that role-playing tends to be a whole lot of fun!

If you are looking to rev things in bed and you want an exciting sex life ahead of you, we recommend the right level of role-playing and sex games. These are the little things that are sure to bring about a change in your sex drive.

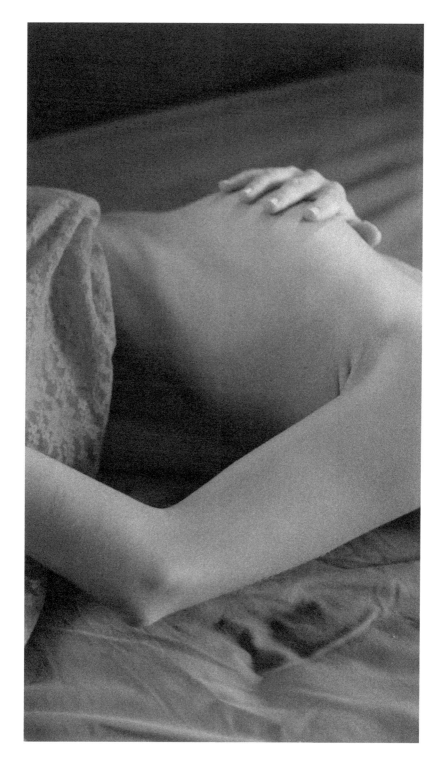

Chapter 2

BDSM Beginner Examples to Try

S exually inspired games are a great way to add more heat to your sex life and build an even stronger level of intimacy with your partner. The games are not ruling but guidelines and suggestions if you are unsure of how to go about them. All the games can be recreated or modified to suit your taste. Some of the games can include light play, costumes, and toys, which can clearly define either a submissive or dominant role or further emphasize a role-playing scenario. Remember always to be able to laugh with your partner during these times, games need not be a serious matter and can also lead to just as pleasing sex without all the extras.

Beginner Games to Try

The games are simple to follow and, of course, easy well suited for the beginner who is tempted to discover more about BDSM and willing to bring more creativity to the bedroom.

A Roll of the Dice

Many online stores and sex shops have a variety of sexually inspired dice. These all hold various body parts, some indicating acts such as kissing or licking, and even sex positions. This a subtle way to mix things up in the bedroom. Toss the dice and follow the instructions, taking turns until you both come to orgasm.

As another option is that you can throw regular dice, depending on the number rolled dictates the number of minutes that your partner needs to go down on you.

BDSM Deck of Cards

Create your own deck of cards with BDSM inspired rewards and punishments. Throw in a few "draw another card" or "double-ups" to keep it interesting.

Draw cards at random or during sex to keep things interesting. You can add new cards to the deck as you come up with new ideas in which to taunt and tease each other.

Orgasm Control

Orgasm control can result in the individual experiencing an ever-stronger orgasm when given a chance. "Edging" is when you control the orgasm of a male specifically. The trick is to bring the person to the edge of orgasm and then stop all forms of stimulation so that they cannot finish. If you find yourself as the submissive, you place your orgasm in the hands of the dominant, which controls the scene and outcome thereof.

The dominant may use their hands, sex toys, or any other form of stimulation to bring you to the peak of orgasm and then stop. A suggestion is to keep doing this until you cannot contain it, the dominant will then take you to orgasm, be prepared for a mind-blowing bed shaking one!

Consider setting an alarm that goes off every minute or so, when this happens, you take turns stimulating each other; this is orgasm control at its best.

Gag Ball

Sex is no longer so much of a taboo as it once was, nor is erotic sex, and many stores sell a selection of gag balls, some of which are beautiful and less threatening. A dominant will use a gag ball to quieten a submissive. As a submissive, it adds a new range of feelings when not able to verbalize what you want.

Pretend that you are in a room full of people and that the aim of the dominant is to make you moan.

Collar

A collar defines the role as a submissive clearly and can be used in specific role-playing scenarios. A dominant might attach a leash to the collar to control the submissive during play.

Question Game

As a submissive, a dominant may ask you a set of questions. For every question you get right, you are rewarded. For every question that you get wrong, you are disciplined.

Rewards can be the following:

- One minute of oral sex

- Two minutes of stimulation with the use of a sex toy or hand

- Three minutes of penetrative sex

- Five minutes of passionate kissing

Discipline can include:

- Orgasm control

- No orgasm, only the dominant is allowed to

- Spanking

- 30 Seconds of nipple clamping

Playing in Public

Playing in public can consist of any acts that make you hot and bothered. It is important to keep in mind how and where you play so as not to break any laws. Public play involves not wearing any underwear, fondling, or even sex in public space such as a restaurant bathroom.

A dominant might also make use of a remote-controlled sex toy, for example, a wireless vibrating bullet. Your pleasure is in your partner's hands, and they determine the intensity and length of the vibrations.

You might also consider taping your sex to enjoy together on another occasion or consider sending nude photos to each other in the middle of a workday.

Task Inspired Games

Tasks are often set out by the dominant for the submissive to complete and are commonplace in BDSM practice.

The point of the game is to set specific, goal-orientated activities for the submissive to try and do within a set time frame, such as making a cup of coffee or collecting something as simple as your handbag or mobile. If they complete the task in time, they are rewarded; if not, they are punished.

A dominant might choose even to distract the submissive, hampering their time to complete the task.

Love Swing

Invest in a door slam love swing that can easily be attached over the top of a closed door. It is bondage-inspired and perfect for couples tempted to try out new sex positions or a bit of BDSM. It is not bulky, nor is it difficult to assemble or disassemble. These swing sets are readily available online. They are adjustable and made to hold roughly 330 lb.

The swing set is great for role-playing, where a submissive takes on the role of somebody being held against their will. Place a mirror in front of the swing to get a birds-eye view of the action.

Role-Playing

It is easy to get stuck in a routine. That is why role-playing is an ideal way in which to bring variety into the bedroom. It also is another characteristic of the BDSM culture and a way in which to establish submissive and dominant roles.

Here are a few ideas to get you in the mood and to get your imagination going:

- Alien and abductee

- Strangers at a bar (Tip, try this at an actual bar or public space.)

- Professor and student

- Explorer and indigenous native

- Master and slave

- Bored housewife and pool boy (or repairman.)

- Sex worker and client

- Pirate and captive

- King and queen

- Kidnapper and the victim

- Photographer and model

- Daddy, daddy

- Fairytale characters

- Animals

The above are just a few examples of how you can bring fantasy elements into the bedroom. There are many other examples and virtually no limitations when it comes to role-playing.

Remember to include extras to your role-playings such as costumes, bondage, blindfolds, and sex toys to enhance the experience further.

Do Not Move

In this game, the submissive is to remain still while the dominant pleases them. If the submissive moves, the dominant can discipline them in the way they see fit. Once the punishment has been issued, the game may continue until the submissive experiences an orgasm.

Follow the Flogger

The submissive is required to keep in contact with the flogger, always. The dominant may set up obstacles to make this harder to achieve. If the submissive breaks, contact with the flogger the dominant is allowed to discipline the submissive via spanking or with the use of the flogger. The game can continue like this until each other's anticipation becomes too great and ends in the bedroom.

Doll Play

The submissive may take on the role of a doll. Role-playing, make-up, and costumes go a long way to achieve this type of play. Just like a toy doll, the dominant may "play" with the doll in any way they would like.

Truth or Dare

When younger truth or dare was always an exciting game to play amongst friends, the aim of the game is simple, ask your partner a series of questions or dares based on sexual encounters or experiences.

For every time that you guess something correctly, your partner may move closer or act on a dare with sexual undertones. As a submissive tied up, this can equal great anticipation depending on the outcome of the dare or correctly or incorrectly answered questions.

Watch a Movie Together

The internet is the most useful tool that you have at your disposal in investigating the weird and rather wonderful world of BDSM. There are many porn sites available, all of which hold a multitude of categories depending on your preference. The idea for this game would be to find a BDSM inspired movie that you could watch together, copying the acts that you see.

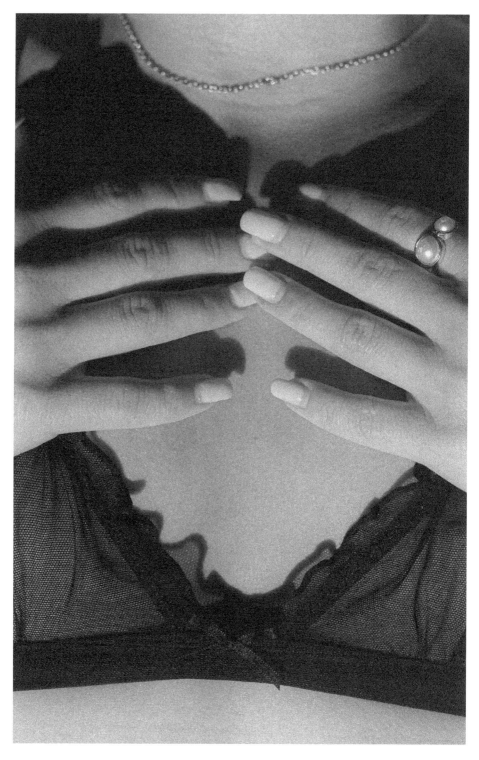

Chapter 3

Anal Sex Guide

D espite the capacity for enjoyment and anticipation, whether it be faith, hygiene, or alleged discomfort for purposes or theories, anal intercourse is hard to deal with. So, let us break a few myths and explore how to think about anal sex before you start a safe conversation about bringing anal sex into your house, so you can prepare to have a "backyard session."

Anal sex is gross. Anal sex is filthy. Although there is a room of germs, likely, given the physiology involved, "no traffic will happen in the pipe." An anal bath and enema may help alleviate the fears of a couple of individuals. It is also necessary to use condoms as frequently as possible and to prevent cross-contamination, given what you may have seen in pornographic films and magazines.

Anal sex is impaired. You can have anal sex as pain-free and fun— if not more— than another kind of gender by following five easy steps to help you relax. Anal sex, because you can get it, is one such part of life that the axiom takes care of what you want. Those who say it will sting will likely be disappointed, and those who fall under the roof will probably be back for a few seconds.

Sexually, your rectum can cause severe permanent damage. Anal intercourse will not permanently damage the rectum if done safely and as an item on your sex list.

When a heterosexual man plays with his ass or asks his girlfriend to do so, he can be homosexual or anal. A heterosexual man cannot make him homosexual any more than he would convert a banana into a monkey using his thumb, tongue, or trick of anal pleasure. Therefore, not all gay men take part in anal sex, and not everyone enjoys bananas. I'll encourage you all to reach into all parts of your body for everyone reading this; maybe you'll have fun like you never had if you were to take the P-spot–your prostate–or get next to it. Trust millions of satisfied hets: Anal playing is not heterosexual— just erotic.

Set the Stage

If you speak about anal sex musically, the soundtrack should be the We Have All Time in the World by Louis Armstrong instead of Bumblebee's Flight by Rimsky-Korsakov. Relax, for in those who wait, good things come. The five notes of anal intercourse are contact, trust, lubricant, breathing, and space. Each of them will optimize the backdoor happiness to you and your family. If you are all gone, you can do the main thing about the pleasure of anal sex: RELAX.

The bedroom is the sexual location preserving and building on knowledge and trust— the two elements that should be present in every sexual relationship.

Take time to make it as easy and worry-free as possible for your bed and your friend. If the penetrated companion distracts and, worst, stupid, he may stop the anal encounter and keep him from returning to a stress-free state.

You should also take the time before starting to wash inside and outside.

When it is "the evening" today, indulge in quickly whatever, that is to suggest, an anal bath or an enema. Anal sex fans are also active in the cleaning process, which contributes to the excitement. Online or from any pharmacy store, you could purchase enamel bags or glasses.

Warm-up: Rub Them the Right Way for Trust and Relaxation

In addition to being necessary for anal sex, the five elements that are required for pleasurable intimacy (communication, trust, lubricants, breathing, time) form an integral part of the traditional tradition of sensuality: massage. Your companion could tell a whole love story with the gentle and caring laying of hands. A massage always stabilizes and calms our body. Because massages are intended to ease us, time and flexibility are needed–a lesson which is also essential for the enjoyment of anal intercourse.

Our hair, rectal flakes, and one of the most excellent all-natural massage lubricants is my favorite sex lubricant: organic coconut oil. Stable at room temperature — "love butter" —and prepared to melt in or on, coconut oil has a tropical-revival scent, and after that movie, it could become your second favorite in your house. The cocoa oil should be scooped into two saucers: one for the pre-game treatment and one for a "main event." Do not scoop directly from the original container for hygienic reasons.

Full-body massages are excellent, but three factors are the better in this example for a backside, the only massage. First, she will be met by the starting position of gender, and therefore we do not aim for the massage to establish intimacy.

Additionally, his sexual thoughts will not be gynocentric as his breasts and vulva remain hidden as she lays on her stomach. Second, the end is in sight with her rear-facing up and right before it. Particularly first face-up massages will lead many to be anxious, as everyone should be calm and ready for what to do. All their vital organs are revealed.

During the treatment, he will take time to realize what his respiration can do by watching and sensing his back rising or sinking beneath his feet. He could straddle her legs with the head facing her to move her back and up, when she exhales, and then encourage her feet, as she inhales, to float gently back to their starting point. He could then massage her arms, thighs, hands, palms, neck, and again to stay as far as practicable from her pussy, partly to make awareness that he is headed straight into Anal Sex, and partly to stop her from dreaming. Be vigilant when massaging her, that she does not tickle; this tightens the hole where she wishes you can relax. Another successful and affectionate way to help her calm is to always put another hand on her because she is face-down and cannot see what he is doing.

He will focus on soothing her and building confidence. It must hold its hands away from the valley between its muscles of two butts until it is prepared for the next step. It might be a smooth, realistic signal to draw a knee towards you or underneath it, showing your fingerprint to your rose.

Now, he should not enter her; however, she welcomes him to touch her bottom. He should instead lubricate his fingers with another coconut oil saucer, which can then end the penetration. She could lay flat and float under her navel a little pillow to raise her rear.

Using his oiled fingertips, he could move his anus around and place light pressure on one of his minor fingers to reach the gap. So, he should not try to get into her as much as she wishes. She is in full control. It works when she reaches out to the rectum as if trying to pull in her hand, to loosen the first sphincter wider. This phase of anal stimulation gives you the opportunity to inject a large quantity of lubricant into the penetrated region. He can put a finger just up to one knuckle and tug and move it so gently while he stays in a method that sounds great to all sensitive newcomers. The game can be used to improve spouse and single sex. I name the game "Tug of Wow."

When she starts calming, even with two fingers in advance, he could switch to a different and similarly well-liked finger and his acceptance. The pair are ready for the next step if they are comfortable, lubricated, and relaxed and know how to regulate the strength of their breath and penetration.

Although this might seem to the penetrator a lot of time, the penetrated individual does need it. If the roles were reversed — a female could enter a person with fingertips or toys (some people call it a street lingo)—men would have empirical evidence that those five measures were necessary for interaction, confidence, respiration, lubricant, and time relaxation. And, ladies, if your partner tells me what a competent and compassionate anal lover you are dating, then I hope that she will be tied with you.

She should feel in control to make a person relax during anal sex. One of the easiest ways to accommodate her penis–and one of the best ways to position her rectum to match her cock–is to get her hands-on top of her.

It helps her to monitor penetration depth and pace, and she can get off quickly every time, very often, when the man's back draws momentum towards his chest, glutes and arms, the blood that must be in his penis. She should be enough to compensate by wrapping her sphincter across her dick, moving away, and relaxing the anal grasp once she lowers onto him.

With anal sex, I urge clients to have antibacterial wipes at hand, and this is the perfect time for them to disinfect their hands while they step backward. The first place goes on with the trust the pair have built up until now, which helps the female to control the penetration depth and speed. It also makes communication between the brain and the ear.

Lie on your back, on a cushion with your face. Stroke yourself as she mounts you to protect your hardon.

Straddle his thighs, toward his mouth. A solution is to put your feet down on either side of his legs if your knees can cope with the pair. You must use your hands for protection if you choose to take this gymnastic pose, or you risk sitting on his penis to wipe away the leverage provided in this position. His cock can easily pass through the first sphincter and avoid the second. If so, take a deep breathe in and move your rectum and on his cock while you are exhaling. Hold this place, if possible, before you feel free. This is an "established" stage of penetration of the anal-penile.

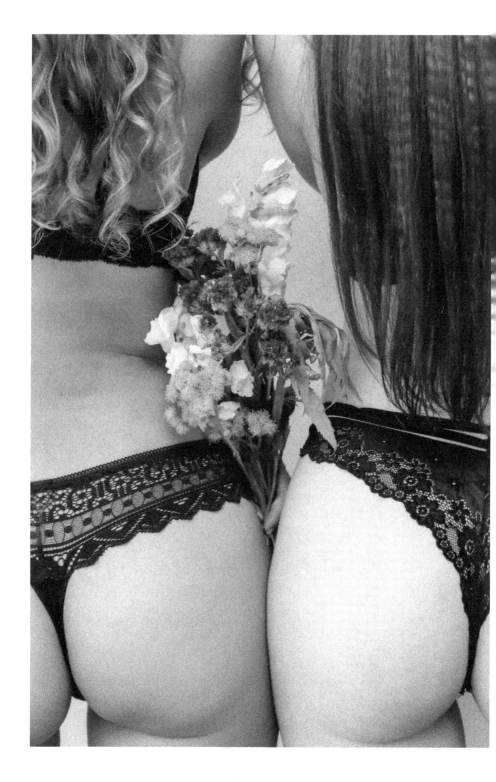

Chapter 4

Anal Sex Tips

I t is defined as the sexual practice during which the penis or an erotic toy is introduced into the anus and the rectum of the partner. Although it was practiced even in Ancient Greece, in our days it is a taboo for many. Some people, in fact, consider it an unnatural act with respect to vaginal coitus. Misinformation in this regard is such that it is considered an exclusive practice of homosexuals and bisexuals, and the benefits or ways in which they are enjoyed are ignored.

Tips in doing Anal Sex

Do not catch a fart before doing it, or do it without planning

This is usually very typical, and I catch a fact that you flip, and apps! accidentally has entered there ... So do not consume psychotropic substances, or get drunk before practicing, this must be planned, discussed by both, and you must agree to try.

Use lubricant

Unfortunately, the anus does not self-lubricate like the vagina, so you must use a good lubricant so that the penetration is not traumatic or painful. Use one that is very dense based on water, and silicone, it will hold you for a long time, and it will be difficult to dry. If you use a condom (which is the most recommended), do not use lubricants with oil, since they end up breaking the latex.

Pornos do not cool to learn

Let's see, watching porn is like watching those short cooking videos that have become fashionable on Facebook, the chef starts doing everything cozily well in a short time, and you're amazed to see how the onions are perfectly cut, all slices appear magically on the table, and nothing gets dirty. In no porn you will see the anal sex preview, you will not see the lubricant, the type that is used, nor will you see the couple talking if they want to try it.

Doing preliminaries: Like a Boss

If preliminary penetration is needed for vaginal penetration, imagine for anal penetration. So, caress the outer part of the anus, while you give pleasure to other sides, lick your partner, cause excitement, in this way you will achieve an erotic connection between the stimuli you receive with anal pleasure. Thus, the receiver will relax and enjoy doing it.

The receiver is the boss

The receiver is to control the depth of penetration, speed, position, and everything! The receiver should be as comfortable as possible to enjoy the experience. It is good that you talk about it beforehand so that afterward you are not shouting the instructions that you should follow while practicing it.

Masturbation during penetration

For girls, it is much better than they masturbate, and stimulate the clitoris while they are penetrated since the nervous system will associate the familiar pleasure with the new experience. This helps a lot to relax and make the moment in general memorable.

Reaching orgasm

The anal orgasm is perfectly achievable by stimulating the G-spot through the buttock. Although it may be a coincidence, since anatomically the G-spot could be in that wall and in others not, this will depend a lot on each person. But fundamentally your partner should be relaxed and should enjoy every sensation. Stress, or nerves, will not help you achieve orgasm.

Change of condom

If you are going to go from anal to vaginal sex, be sure to change the condom or clean yourself very well since you can transmit bacteria and cause serious infections such as UTI. Do not exaggerate with the lubricant, so that it does not run everywhere, this can also cause infections.

Squeeze a lot, and ejaculate quickly?

If you suffer from premature ejaculation, explains Charlie Glickman, sex educator, and author of The Ultimate Guide to Prostate Pleasure , do not use numbing creams under any circumstances: "It is like you're going to remove a tooth, and the dentist will inject Novocain, and when you go to eat you do not feel the face. " It is understood that this should be enjoyed, so you can use condoms retardants, or look for information on how to avoid premature ejaculation.

Why is it a pleasant activity?

Anal penetration offers great pleasure since during the act the clitoris is stimulated by the rectum up to the pelvic area.

In psychological terms, then, prohibited acts become aphrodisiacs. This is because it is a practice considered new, which makes it even more excited. Anatomically, in addition, the anal area contains a large amount of touch-sensitive nerve fibers.

Lubricating the Area

The anus does not naturally lubricate during sexual intercourse like the vagina. Consequently, it is essential to carry out penetration with precaution, in fact, the muscles of this area do not enjoy the same elasticity.

The use of the lubricant is essential; it is also possible to lubricate the area naturally with saliva. In any case, the effect ends soon, so you do not have to wait long before entering.

Anal Simulation

The ideal is a combination of penetration and masturbation, as it increases pleasure and relaxes the muscles.

After deciding to have anal sex, you must abandon the prejudices. Anal coitus is not only a physical emotion but also a subjective one.

Does anal masturbation exist? Yes, it is a method by which one or more fingers are introduced and genital manipulation is performed at the same time. This prevents injury to the walls of the rectum.

What is the Cause of the pain?

When the act is done quickly, the muscles are not relaxed, and the sphincter is closed. Therefore, anal sex is painful. It is therefore advisable to follow the various steps carefully.

How to do it?

- First, it is possible to dilate the anal sphincter with the help of a water-based lubricant

- Then a finger is slowly introduced into the anus by gentle movements

- The goal is to expand it to sufficient expansion progressively

- Finally, penetration is realized

It is the only way to avoid pain.

Hygiene and Safety

The mucosa covering the rectal area is prone to contracting infections and injuries, in the worst case, an anal fissure. For this reason, we recommend the following:

- Hurried penetration causes breaks that produce bleeding and injuries

- These, in turn, facilitate the appearance of sexually transmitted diseases such as herpes, gonorrhea or syphilis. The use of condoms is mandatory

- The idea is to wash before and after penetration

- You must have short nails

- One of the most frequent fears is that during the act an incident with feces occurs. In this case, it is possible to make an enema that helps clean the rectum

Benefits for Women When Practicing Anal Sex

Without unwanted dwarves

The risk of getting pregnant if they give you back is practically nil, if not impossible. This is one of the main reasons for letting your boy give you from behind because you will not leave with the typical surprises like "he has not let me down".

Help release tension.

Even if you do not believe it, practicing it for the "little one" can relax as never if it is done with care, because when the man "goes through Detroit" stimulates certain nerve endings that women have there, they help release hormones that relax the body

Natural painkiller

Forget about having to use medication every time you have a headache, muscle or cramps of the period, because thanks to the endorphins and oxytocin that are released when you start to enjoy doing it out there, they have an amazing analgesic effect that helps relieve the pain.

Rejuvenator

In addition to helping to release tensions, the "litter" inside the an can be very beneficial, since the semen helps to observe the selenium that is in it, reducing wrinkles and increasing the years of life.

Reinforced relationship

If you do it, your boy will know that he can trust 100% in you because you are giving him something that perhaps you have not given anyone else, this will help strengthen the relationship between the two. No doubt you should do it immediately.

Chapter 5

First Time Lesbian Sex Guide and

What to Expect

Finding Your Ideal Partner

Here is the main place that your situation will factor into finding the partner you seek. While many bi-curious women would love to experience an encounter with someone who is far more experienced, the truth of the matter is that the majority of lesbians will be offended if they are being used "as an experiment".

In a situation where you are seeking a threesome with your man, this is especially true. Any woman who identifies as a lesbian will be utterly insulted if you ask her to join in with you and your boyfriend or husband. Similarly, many will refuse to be the action on the side with someone who is in a committed relationship with a man, although some are willing to negotiate if all parties involved are aware of the situation. This varies from woman to woman, however, and it is imperative that you be honest with your potential partner to ensure that no one gets hurt. Ideally, you should seek another woman who is either bisexual or bi-curious.

If you are not involved in a heterosexual relationship, but you are not certain if you are truly attracted to women or just curious, it may be best to seek a partner who is also curious. This may be a good opportunity to join a couple that is looking for a "third", if you are interested in this experience. However, there may be less pressure if you choose to have a one-on-one experience with someone at the same level as yourself. When the parties involved are at similar experience levels, neither will feel intimidated or pressured into a stellar performance.

For our small fourth category, we are going to operate under the assumption that you have already found the partner you seek your first sexual activity with, but you are not sure how to proceed. Just as in any other sexual relationship, it can be tough to understand how to move forward, particularly when you do not already have the experience of success behind you. Rest assured, although you may feel that you are alone, you most certainly are not.

No matter which of these categories you fall in, the primary consideration is that there is no reason to lie. If you are truthful about your pursuits, you will find the woman who is just right for your first experience.

Where to Look

If you already have your partner, feel free to skip this step. For those of you who are still looking, however, you need to evaluate what you want out of this experience. If you are seeking a strictly sexual experience, your options are much wider than someone who is looking for a romantic relationship with an implied sexual aspect.

There is a joke among the gay community that "dating [for us] is like looking for a job; you either need a referral or you do it online." It is true, though; since many people are not interested in the same sex, it can be difficult to find someone to hook up with.

Option #1: Check the Internet. This can be simple, as there are numerous dating sites available, and most of them are both free and accommodating to "alternative" lifestyles. You must be careful when browsing online for a date, however, as there is always some degree of risk involved with meeting someone this way. All it takes is a simple Internet search to turn up a myriad of options. Be sure to let the women you speak to know of your intentions; that is, if you are seeking a purely sexual relationship or one with a romantic connotation as well.

If you decide to use the Internet, you must be incredibly careful. I recommend you tell someone (who is local enough to be helpful to you) where you will be and who you will be meeting with. You do not have to tell them that you are planning to get lucky, but they should know that you are meeting someone so that you have a safety net.

Option #2: Find an LGBTQ gathering. This can include "pride" clubs at your local college or university, pride rallies and parades, meet-ups, and even some church groups. While the basic idea of most of these venues is to network, rather than to find love and sex, that is not to say that it cannot happen. Keep your expectations low, and allow yourself to make friends, first and foremost. These friends can be useful for

Option #3, listed below. If you are old enough, you can choose to hit the bars as well, although this is not really the greatest option as alcohol can hinder your decision-making process and is not supported by all cultures. However, it remains an option for those who are legally allowed and personally inclined to do so.

Option #3: Ask around. This is probably a last resort for your first time, as telling your friends and family that you want to have sex with a woman can be tough to work around. However, if you have friends who you know are cool with the gay community, it does not hurt to ask if they know someone! It is even possible that they will offer their services. This would, of course, be the safest option, because the woman would already have an established chemistry with you, and you would know that you were in safe hands. However, generally, people are shy about their first time, and this can be an embarrassing question.

What to Expect

You need to exude confidence, even if you must fake it. This is ultimately more important than the skill you may or may not have. (Certainly, some women are just "cut out" for it, but many others must learn through doing.) You need to concentrate on how much you want this and let that guide you.

If you are more aroused by the sight of her naked body, it is time to press forward. Begin by caressing her skin. Think of the places on your body that get you wet when touched (if you have experience with heterosexual activities). The most common spots may be her sides, her butt, and her legs – do not neglect these! Make sure you explore other areas, also; every woman has her own erogenous zones that provide her with the necessary stimulation.

If your partner is willing to be penetrated, feel free to slide one or two fingers in her. If she has been penetrated before, most likely two fingers will provide the perfect size for her pleasure, but if it seems a little too tight, you should start with one. You do not want to hurt her, after all. Despite what you may think, thrusting is not as important for lesbian sex – in fact, a wiggling motion is much more effective. (Think of how you would signal someone over to you; this is basically the motion you will want to use.) Once your fingers are inside of her, you should be able to feel the G-spot. Gentle pressure in this area can work wonders!

If you would like (and she is accepting), you can also go down on her at this point. Gently kissing the area is a good place to start. Let your intuition (and your partner's communication!) guide you here. Even if you have never really considered the idea before, you will have some sense of what to do based on your own arousal and your partner's instruction. (Believe me, she will guide you.)

The rest is up to you. Although there is a common myth among the lesbian community that "girls know what girls like", the truth is, and every woman is different. What turns one on may completely turn off another, and the only way to truly learn is to try. Chances are, you will find things that work, and things that do not. It is all part of the learning process.

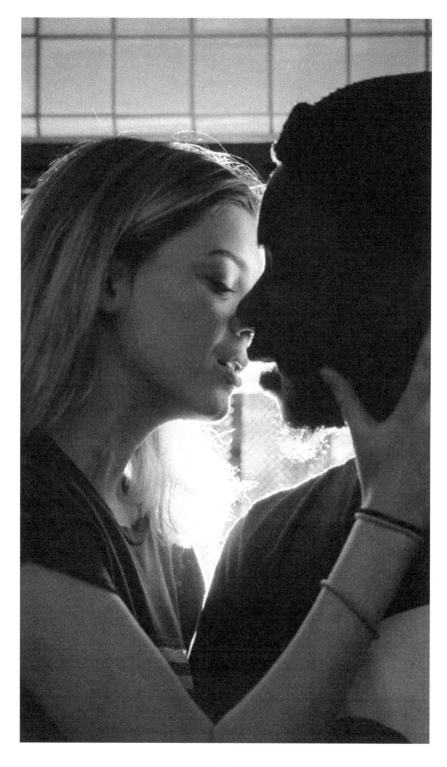

Chapter 6

Advanced Orgasms

The Orgasm

For a woman to reach orgasm, much of this is dependent on her mindset. She will need to feel comfortable being vulnerable in this space for her to reach her full arousal potential. She needs to reach this point for her to orgasm and in order for her to enjoy sex fully. For this reason, mindset and pleasure are very closely linked to a woman.

The Clitoral Orgasm

When the clitoris is rubbed in the right way, it will lead to orgasm, just like the penis of a man. Treating it like this can give both men and women insight into how it works and how to make the woman come. When stimulated physically with someone's fingers or a sex toy like a vibrator, this can lead to an orgasm for the woman. The clitoris is a structure that contains many nerve endings, which is what makes it so sensitive. When a woman is not aroused sexually, her clitoris is still there, but it will not be as enlarged as when she is horny.

Vaginal Pleasure

A woman's vagina automatically swells when she is sexually aroused because of increased blood flow to her genitals, sort of like how your penis becomes erect when you get horny. What this means for you is that when your penis is inside of her, the walls of her vagina will tighten and swell as the blood flow increases, and you will feel this effect on your penis, resulting in added pleasure for you.

Multiple Orgasms

There are different types of multiple orgasms that a woman can achieve. Women are lucky in that they can have both back-to-back orgasms and blended orgasms. They are even able to have back-to-back blended orgasms in some cases! We will learn more about the different types of multiple orgasms.

Blended Orgasms

A blended orgasm is achieved when multiple different orgasms are achieved at the same time. This can be two different orgasms at the same time, or in some cases, even more than two! This type of orgasm leads to even more pleasure than a single orgasm and will lead the woman to feel more intense pleasure than ever before. During penetration, there is lots of opportunity for different types of female orgasms to occur. The two most common ways that a woman can reach orgasm are through her clitoris and through her G-spot. We will look at some ways that a woman can have both orgasms at the same time, as well as some other options for blended orgasms.

Any combination of these separate but simultaneous orgasms compound to give the woman a mind-blowing, full-body, blended orgasm, this is especially so if the two locations of stimulation are a larger distance from each other- like the nipples and the clitoris, for example. The best type of blended orgasm will vary from woman to woman, depending on her personal preferences and what her most sensitive erogenous zones are. Some of these zones include the clitoris, the anus, the G-Spot, and the nipples. Some women may have others as well, but this is largely dependent on the woman's body.

Clitoral and G-Spot Blended Orgasm

The first method is a clitoral orgasm during penetration. If the clitoris is stimulated while the man is penetrating the woman, it is possible that she can have an orgasm through both her clitoris and her G-Spot at the same time. This type of multiple orgasm will make her feel pleasure like never because these two places are extremely pleasurable even when achieved alone, so together, it is a new level of orgasm! There are different ways that you can achieve this, but the most successful way is to penetrate her with your fingers while she rubs her clitoris at the same time. This way, you can feel your way around and stimulate her G-spot while she pleases herself. It may take some practice and will require a lot of communication, but eventually, you will both be able to time it so that she can have both orgasms at once. Another way that this can happen is while the man is thrusting his penis into her. While he is doing this, she can touch her clitoris using her fingers or a vibrator, or the man can stimulate her clitoris by using his fingers or a vibrator. Some specific positions will allow for the man's penis to reach the G-Spot when inside of her, and at the same time, the base of his penis or his pelvic region can rub her clitoris, causing both orgasms to happen at the same time.

Anal and Clitoral Blended Orgasm

Another way that a woman can achieve a blended orgasm is through having both an anal and a clitoral orgasm at the same time. This is like the blended orgasm in which the man is penetrating the woman with his penis. At the same time, her clitoris is being stimulated, but in this case, it is done while you are having anal sex. The method will happen in a similar way to the vaginal penetration with clitoral stimulation, but the positions used will be slightly different as the positions used in this case would be ones that better allow for anal penetration while giving either the man or the woman free hands to stimulate the clitoris. Either the man or the woman can stimulate the woman's clitoris in a variety of anal sex positions using either their hands or a vibrating sex toy.

Back-to-Back Orgasms

Not only can women have blended orgasms, but they can also have back-to-back orgasms. These orgasms occur one after the other and give the woman immense pleasure because she can keep coming again and again and again.

This type of repeated orgasm is only possible for women as the male body is unable to do this. This is since the male body has to wait for a refractory period after every orgasm. What this means is that there is an amount of time after an orgasm during which a man's body is unable to achieve an erection or have another orgasm. During this time, his body is recovering from the orgasm and needs this time to recuperate. The length of this period is different for every man, but it ranges between fifteen to thirty minutes in most males.

The great thing about the clitoris is that after orgasm, it may be very sensitive for a few minutes, but it maintains its "erection" and can be stimulated again a very short time after for a doubly pleasurable second orgasm. This can lead to a third and a fourth and beyond. Therefore, it is beneficial to give a woman an orgasm during foreplay as it will increase her chances of orgasm during penetration because of how horny it will have made her. Sometimes, women's pleasure only builds after an initial orgasm instead of going back to zero before climbing again like a man's pleasure would have to.

It is important for men to understand this difference because they can then take advantage of it and pleasure their woman to the fullest. While they await their refractory period, they can please their woman in a way that does not involve their penis, give her an orgasm, and then by the time this happens. He will be ready to get hard again and have a second round with her. All the while, she will become increasingly horny and pleased.

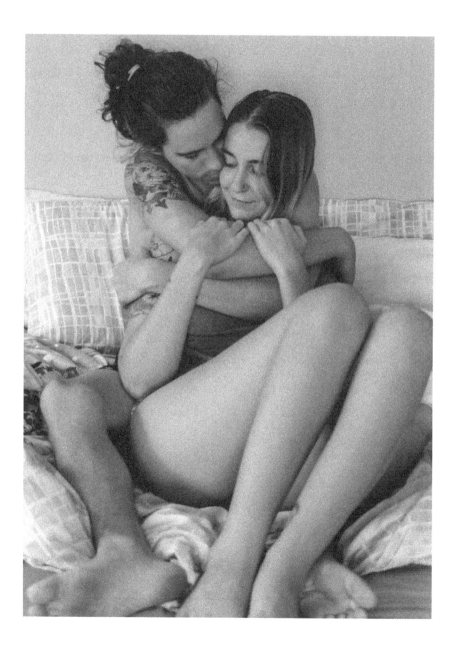

Chapter 7

Bisexual

Okay so where is the number one place to look for it? It is Craigslist there are 100's of daily ads of men looking for gay sex. I filter it for pictures as you like to see a picture of the cock you will be sucking that day. See how easy it is? Imagine it this easy with a woman? No way! With a guy, you know you are going to get laid and lay someone. The possibilities are endless. You will have no problem finding a man's cock to suck or some dude blowing your cock. You can probably meet at least one dude a day to suck off, maybe two depending how frisky you are Now, I will tell you about my first sexual encounter I had on Craigslist. My first was with a 34-year-old white dude named James. How it all came about was I just broken up with my girlfriend who cheated on me, so feeling stressed out one night and horny I decided I wanted to get laid, so I went on Craigslist seeking a woman.

For my first encounter, I wanted a man who was kind of like me a pale white Irish dude. Looking around the ad I noticed this dude name James who had this huge white cock. He said in his ad he like to suck cock. So, as I was hesitant at first, but we than exchanged pictures. Remember at first, I wanted just my cocked sucked, but the seeds had been planted in my mind that maybe just this once I will try sucking on a cock...

So, we exchange phone numbers and talk. He seems like a friendly fellow and we decide to meet at a cheap motel. I get there first and put the rom in my name. I head upstairs, then James phones me he has arrived. I tell him what room I am in, and excitedly wait for him. Knock on my door. I open it and the first thing I notice is his deep penetrating blue eyes. We exchange a strong handshake, and a few hellos. We start my talking about what we like such as sports, music, and video games. We are both nervous and excited. I tell James this is my first time, and he tells me it is his first time as well.

To break the tensions, I break out some beer and wine coolers. This drinking last about a good twenty minutes, then I say ok let`s get it on. I grabbed him by the head, and start to kiss him on the lips, and then he starts to lick my neck below my ear. I am surprised how good it feels. He then starts to nibble on my neck which excites me as a I get boner. I than return the favor by licking his neck, we both now start to get on the bed. I unzip his pants, while he unzips mine. We go into a 69 position. He starts to suck my cock. I love it, now I try cock for the first time. I put James cock in my mouth. It tastes good. All these years I wonder what a cock would taste like, and I am happy to report it tastes good. We now suck away. It is like an animal instinct in me took over. I continue to suck his cock like I never sucked anything before. I noticed his cock keep getting bigger in my mouth. We continue go back n forth, we both start calling each other derogatory names, and for some reason it turns me on. I call him a faggot, and he calls me a cocksucker. The more we call each other names the harder I get, then I cum all over his face. I just exploded. What a rush. Now I take cock a keep sucking it. I want him to cum I want to taste it, then boom he shoots a load, and I just licked it up. Wow! This was so intense. I loved it. His cum also tasted good, and now I know why women suck cock. That was it. We talk, and exchange numbers.

Another place to find gay sex is Grindr.

One day I was driving along, and I felt horny. I was going to call James, but I knew he was working, So I was in a dilemma, also I for some reason wanted to try a black cock. I heard the place to find black cock quick was the app Grindr you find on your smart phone. Grindr is cool in that you just swipe it and see if some dude wants to hook up with you. How easy is that? Well, I found this black guy on their named Devin who was looking for a quick blowjob in a car This was so cool because instead of renting out a motel we could drive our cars next to each other and suck each other off quick! So, Devin and I made plans to drive our cars to a wooded area near a truck stop. I showed up first, then Devin showed up with his powerful BLACK SPORTS CAR. He was good looking. A six pack, tight ass, and dreads. He got into my car, and he slowly went down on me. It was so exciting to let him blow me out in the woods. I blew a load quick in his mouth, now the moment I always fantasied about was here. I was going to suck my first black cock.

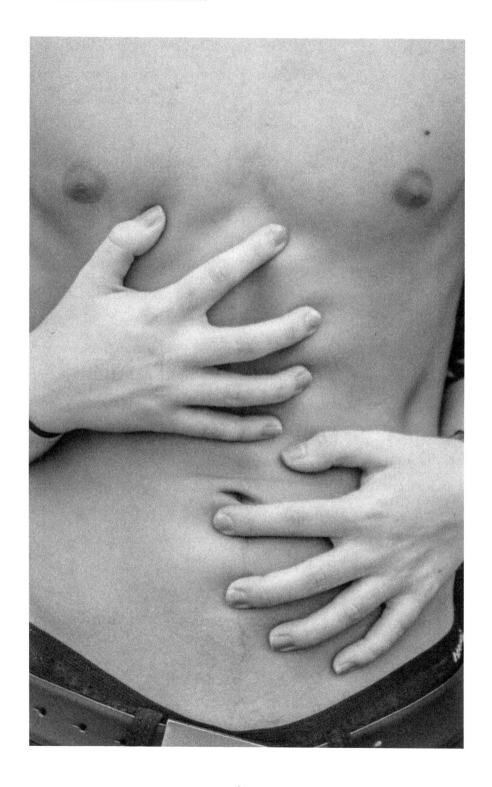

Chapter 8

Everybody's Different

Most of us have had reasonably varied sex lives, as modern people. Few of us come to marriage, or long-term partnerships as virgins, unless we are either very young, or very cloistered. So, it is clear that most modern adults know what it is like to have sexual experiences that are disappointing and unsatisfying. It is inevitable that this should happen when we approach sex as a sport, a diversion, or something to be pursued with little thought as to the spiritual nature of our sex partners. What could be more disappointing than sex that did not make us feel connected to our partners?

But there are times when physical realities beyond anyone's control are what get in the way of satisfying sex. Sometimes, we end up in bed with people to whom we are not well-matched, physically. If we truly care about someone, we find our way around these physical realities. Interestingly, the Kama Sutra has a prescription for the physical statuses of men and women and about who fits best with whom. I am sure you will agree, after reading through the physical types laid out in Kama Sutra, that there is some logic involved. But our brief must be read in the light of the sexual advice offered to mitigate the disparities described in terms of male/female genitalia.

Physical Types

Kama Sutra sets out three categories of both men and women, concerning the various characteristics of their respective genitalia. I trust no one will personalize any of what is to follow. We are made the way we are made and (amazingly), one size does not fit all! In fact, there are physical types to which we are more suited than others, according to Kama Sutra. We all know how it feels to find a lover who "fits". We also know how to accommodate lovers who fit a little less perfect, through experience and the application of emotional tenderness and attachment.

Men are classified as hares, bulls, or horses. I do not suppose anyone will have too much difficulty discerning what we are talking about here. We are talking about the size of what is called in the Kama Sutra the "lingam" (male genitalia). Of the three types, hares are the smallest and horses, the largest.

Women are classified as deer, hares, or elephants. These designations refer to the "yoni" (female genitalia) and refer specifically to depth. In Kama Sutra, the largest male size corresponds to the medium size in the female. In fact, the Kama Sutra posits that the male member determines the level of satisfaction in the female by being a little "too much". Many women will attest that size does not matter. This is, in fact, not only a bromide to soothe the frayed ego of males of smaller genital dimensions. It is true. The male member is only as good as its host's expertise. While the Kama Sutra doesn't mention this aspect of sexuality, I'd be more than willing to go out on a limb and guess that the information offered concerning sexual congress is (at least to some extent) intended to mitigate the effect of "mismatched" genitalia.

Suffice to say that the physical typology of Kama Sutra, while an interesting artifact of the times it was written in, perhaps reflects a truth about the male authors that most women will readily recognize. Women know that the size of the lingam pales in importance next to the sexual expertise of their lovers. For this reason, it is important to read Kama Sutra in its setting and take from it that speaks most eloquently to us and our times.

Whether you are a hare, a deer, an elephant, or a horse, the appropriateness and harmony of your match has much more to do with your approach and interplay with your partner than it does with the size of your genitalia. I believe this assessment is more than fair and serves to soften perhaps the blow of the somewhat arbitrary genital typology offered in the Kama Sutra.

Levels of Passion (Libido)

We all have varying levels of need for sexual union. Even between loving partners, these levels can be at odds with one another. They are not static, though. Our libidos wax and wane, as part of the rhythms of our lives. There will be times when we are either both more inclined to our sexualities, less so inclined, or when we are at opposite ends of our respective libidinous arcs. The Kama Sutra also describes the various levels of passion and how they can be manifested in our sex lives.

Some people seem to have an endless amount of sexual energy. Others, very little. They tend to believe that sex is not all that important. Others are between these two polarities. The Kama Sutra states that both men and women can fall into any of these three categories: intense, weak, and middling, its further states that some go for the long game, others are satisfied in very little time and still others are of mediocre endurance. But the Kama Sutra all makes special provision for the very specific needs of women and puts them in the driver's seat in terms of sexual endurance.

Because women (for the most part) do not ejaculate in the same way men do, women take an entirely different approach to sexuality. This is, in fact, the model. During lovemaking, women feel pleasure as a more holistic experience, whereas men tend to focus on intercourse and the finality of their own orgasms. Because of this key sexual difference, women can reach climax, but continue to be connected to their partners physically and entirely invested in continuing the experience. Men, having reached ejaculation, tend to disconnect entirely – even fall asleep! This can be a bit of a problem for women who are interested in continuing the sexual encounter, once the man they are with ejaculates, rolls over the goes to sleep.

There is a biological reason for this male habit, one supposes, but it certainly does not serve the needs of the woman, which are paramount in the realm of making love.

The Kama Sutra's explanation for this variance between men and women is, once again, a product of the time in which it was written. There was little in the way of biological information available to people in those times. And so, the Kama Sutra tends to cast the woman as emitting "semen" from beginning to end of any given lovemaking session. Of course, as modern people with access to information the ancients had no knowledge of, we know this is not the case. All the same, it might have seemed a good explanation at the time, as men attempted to unravel the mysteries of the feminine.

It is for this reason that the Kama Sutra counsels sexual continence. This method sees the male withholding his own orgasm for the sake of prolonged lovemaking, in order that the highest quality of sexual union is reached. Women, the notes, can be satisfied without a great investment of time, but this is not the desired type of sexual union. A truly transcendent sexual experience is prolonged, unhurried, and exploratory in a highly sensual way. Sexual continence serves those seeking this type of sexual experience, as it calls on the man to be attentive to the quality of sex he is sharing with his partner and to put aside the need to climax.

Chapter 9

Lubricants, Gels, Toys, and their Role

Lubes can sometimes be essential. The vagina can sometimes fail to self-lubricate enough for both of you to enjoy the intercourse session. Lubricants and gels are especially necessary whenever you are getting into anal penetration, simply because the ass is not capable of self-lubricating like the vagina.

In a nutshell, lubricants have sex more enjoyable and comfortable. The juices excreted by the vagina and saliva will not give sufficient lubrication to get the job done correctly. Even if you have some alone time and feel the mood to masturbate, whether it is with your hand or using tools, lubricants will help take your experience to a whole other level.

You need to have in mind that you cannot just use any lubricant or gel you find; you need to get one that is explicitly made for sexual intercourse. You can find a wide array of lubes in many drug stores and in any sex shop you can find. Technology has made buying lubes even more convenient because you can order online from the comfort of your home and have it delivered to you; in some cases, delivery can be made within the hour!!

There are two main types of lubricants and gels that are available in the market, both of which come in various brands and scents.

Water-Based Lubricants and Gels

One quality of water-based lubricants that makes them the preferred choice of many is that they do not easily stain and cleaning them up is quite easy. They are also available in a wide array of tastes, textures, ingredients, and consistencies. These lubricants are also very much compatible with all the materials used to have sex toys, as well as those that are used to manufacture both latex and non-latex condoms.

You need to note, however, that the majority percentage of these water-based lubricants are manufactured using glycerin, and this can make some people uncomfortable or even cause problems. Many women attributes glycerin to be the cause of an imbalance in the yeast levels in their vagina and also yeast infections. This, however, does not affect anal sex, and therefore the preference for most people having the lube, which does not contain glycerin to avoid unnecessary problems. When it comes to anal sex, there are some people who find that lubricants that contain high levels of glycerin tend to stimulate their bowel movements and prefer to avoid them when engaging in anal sex. No need to worry though, there is an increase in the number of lubricants that do not contain any glycerin, and also there are some that do not even contain paraben.

In terms of consistency, water-based lubricants completely cover that scale. They are available in varying levels of liquidity, ranging from super-thick, thick, medium, and thin. Any lubricant can greatly facilitate penetration, but thick and super-thick lubricants are better suited for anal penetration. The reason is that they possess a consistency that is very similar to hair gel. They tend lasting longer and protect the gentle rectal tissue by acting as a cushioning layer.

Depending on your preferences, if you always prefer to put either your hands, sec toys, or even a penis in your mouth after they have come in contact with a lubricant or gel, you might want to purchase a lubricant that has a pleasant taste, or at least, a flavor that you can stand. Some water-based lubricants taste of chemicals or have a sour taste that is a significant turn-off. There are quite a number of sexual lubricants on the market that are flavored, and if you are not lucky enough to find your taste of choice in the first attempt, you may have to taste quite a number of flavors.

Among the current trends as far as water-based lubricants are concerned is warming lubricants. These lubricants create a warming effect upon contact. There are, however, various ingredients, and they are:

- Acacia honey or any of its derivatives (Astroglide warming liquid, wet warming lubricant, and KY warming liquid)

- Menthol (hot elbow grease, liquid sizzle that is glycerin free, and ID sensation)

☐   Cinnamon back (emerita OH). It is the most natural among them all.

The honey or menthol generates a warming feeling that makes blood rush to the genitals, thereby assisting in the arousal process.

As far as lubricants are concerned, whether you like, it depends on your personal preferences and what you find comfortable. Some people believe that they love the way it causes their private parts to tingle; others have horror stories about them (probably did not know about the glycerin). A vast majority of women prefer warming lubricants because they have an element of protecting the vagina, but at the same time, many people find that they get an overwhelming feeling whenever they use this warming lubricant for anal penetration.

Silicon-Based Lubricants

Lubricants and gels that are made using silicon are quickly becoming popular among its users. Some brands that have silicone-based lubricants and gels include System JO Original, ID Velvet, Swiss Navy Silicon, Eros gel, Wet platinum, and KY Intrigue. Just like water-based gels and lubricants, silicon-based lubes are also do not stain. They, however, are odorless and are more expensive than water-based lubricants and gels because they do not dry up as fast (they last longer), and therefore you only use less lube.

Silicon gels are usually more concentrated and, therefore, can go a long way. A lot of people typically have a liking to silicon's slick texture and its fantastic quality of not being sticky or even tacky like their water-based counterparts. Some people claim that this sleek texture of silicon has a lot of friction, making it a better option for anal sex.

Silicon-based lubricants work well with both latex condoms and non-latex condoms and other safe sex barriers, a select number of materials used to have sex toys including glass, rubber, metal, and hard plastic. Sex toys that are made using silicon are entirely incompatible with silicon-based gels and lubricants as they get damaged. The only way that silicon sex toy lovers can get to lubricate them with silicon-based lubricants and gels is by wrapping them up with a condom. If you like to get a little freaky in the shower or a swimming pool, silicon-based lubes and gels are the best option because, unlike water-based lubricants, they remain slick underwater. This quality makes them the best choice of getting the job done in such scenarios.

Oil-Based Lubricants and Gels

Oil-based gels and lubricants and those that are vegetable-based, whether you bought them or common household goods such as petroleum jelly, baby oil, or even lotions, are not recommended. The simple reason behind this is that they are very messy and leave behind nasty stains on whatever they encounter. They are also responsible for the breakage of latex condoms and the pieced sex dolls.

The most significant risk that these lubes have is that these lubes, and gels have a tendency of setting camp inside the vagina, and they cannot get flushed out of the body. This is very unhealthy to the woman because it becomes a perfect spot where bacteria can breed, and this will eventually result in a vaginal infection. Even if you use these lubes for anal sex, they always make their way to the vagina, and the result is the same. The best thing you can do to spice up your sex life is using oil and vegetable-based lubricants for their intended purpose, not sex. Men can, however, use them for masturbation, but make sure to rinse off your penis thoroughly before you can penetrate someone else.

How to Properly Use Lubricants and Gels

Using lubricants and gels is a straightforward process. You need to apply it on whatever you need to insert, be it a penis, finger, or a sex toy, then slide it in. You need to remember that water-based lubricants and gels dry up quicker, and therefore you should use a lot of it and be prepared to refill it halfway through. Silicon-based lubes do not dry up quickly, and therefore you can comfortably use it sparingly. You can have it around, though, to keep it spicy. A box of baby wipes or pocket tissues can also come in handy to wipe out any extra gel, spillages, or any other accidents that may occur.

Sex Toys

The vulva contains exterior lips, internal lips, scissors, frenuls, and openings of the urethra, the clitoral hood, and the clitoral glans. The vulva comprises the outside labia. Many people describe the vagina throughout the entire genital area, but that is incorrect. The word Vulva and one I use in the entire novel is right. Outer lips are the internal lips of the vulva (also known as the labia majora). We have hair follicles and are, of course, rugged. You can brush, touch, kiss and even twitter them softly, and the internal labia are receptive. Within lips are the two hairless central lips of the vulva (also known as labia minora). It can be slim or small, wide, and thin, one of them or somewhere between them. The inner lips are more sensitive than the external lips. They burst in color when a wife is turned on. It is important to know that the vulva of every person is different: some have big external lips, and some have small internal lips that are more prominent than their outer lips. Many lips of women are similar in size, some of the asymmetric. A sensitive area is a tissue where the internal lips touch on the bottom of the spoon. The skin with its inner lips at the top is the frenulum, and many females, especially as this position is near to the clitoral gland and cap, may be very responsive.

Chapter 10

How to Prepare Your Mind and Body for Sex

The secret to an invigorating sex life lies within the mind. Do you remember when sex seemed like a seven-course feast? You did not know what was coming. Next, every mouthful made you tingle from head to toe, and once you reached the end of it, you felt content and satisfied. Nowadays, it seems like a bowl of cereal, convenient, quick, and fills a gap, but it is not something you would want to have every single day.

To get great sex back, you need to put it on the brain. When you make sure that you turn your brain on before you have sex, it will trigger your libido. Let us take a moment to look at some ways to get your mind ready for sex.

Take it Slow

How come a man can go from watching a slasher film to hopping into bed and instantly feeling horny, but a woman hops into bed and starts to think about everything they must do the next day? The female brain and the male brain work differently. A woman's brain works by multitasking, but a man's brain typically focuses on one thing at a time.

Just Say Yes

For some, having sex can be like having to go to the gym. Their body and mind start to rebel against it, but once they do, they feel great. Standard wisdom has said, for a woman, the sexual cycle goes from desire to arousal to orgasm. There has been new research that has found that women who are in long-term relationships will experience desire after they become aroused. That means, sometimes, you simply must be receptive to your partner's touch instead of giving in to the voice that is telling you to go to sleep.

When you give into that touch, your brain will start to focus on pleasures that follow and will then increase the blood flow to the right areas. Even if all you have is a quickie and you do not orgasm, the bio chemicals released during sex are still released, which will help you to want to have more sex, more often.

There are ways for women to help get themself aroused instead of waiting on their partners to initiate. You can start by tensing your pelvic floor muscles. All of these muscles support your pelvic floor, as well as your genitals, and helps to stimulate the arousal process.

Fantasy

You can also use your mind to help trigger desire for your partner. There is a simple exercise you can do for this. You and your partner sit across from one another, hold hands, and then stare into one another's eyes. Do not say a word, but both of you should start to think about the last time that you had sex and enjoyed it. This helps to create a connection between the mind and body. It works a lot like how you shiver when you recall a scary experience. When focusing on all the little sexy details, it will ignite your body and turn you on. You will also get to see the arousal on your partner's face.

Get Some Sleep

There is nothing worse than falling asleep before sex. One of the main reasons why new parents lose their sex lives is that they are too tired. Sex just does not sound good when you have not had enough sleep. If you have noticed that you are too tired to get intimate, you need to make sure that you make sleep a priority. Make sure that you are getting the recommended seven to nine hours each night. To improve your sleep, you should make sure all devices are turned off.

Food

We know a healthy diet is important for a long and healthy life, but the foods you eat can also affect your libido. Foods like honey, peanut butter, and bananas contain vitamin B, which naturally boosts your libido. Celery contains androsterone, which can help aid in female attraction. There are a lot of other foods out there that act as natural aphrodisiacs as well.

Understand Her Cycle

Women are influenced by their cycle. They will find sex more enjoyable at different times of their cycle. From day one to 14, women produce more testosterone, which means it is easier to get turned on and reach climax. Women also experience a surge in libido during days 24 to 28 because of the nerve endings that are stimulated by the thickening of the uterine lining.

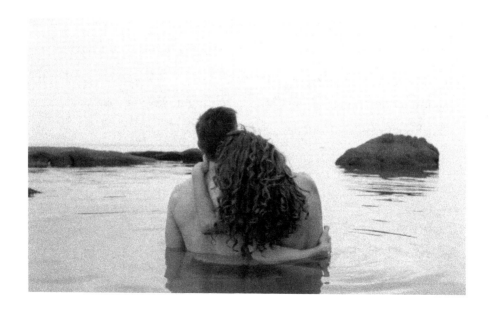

Chapter 11

G-spot Stimulating Sex Positions

For a sex position to feel amazing then it must be hitting the most sensual spots for both the man and woman and this is when we should believe the heat is on the G-spot. We are getting it right because intense pleasure and multiple orgasm is eminent. The truth is that there are sex positions that can easily stimulate this spot and help give unimaginable pleasures. So, if you want to drive your partner crazy and hit the G-spot for more stimulation, then you need to check out these 10 sultry sex positions that will help you achieve your aim.

· **The Wheelbarrow Sex Position**

The wheelbarrow sex position is one position that gets both partners screaming and moaning to the clouds. You cannot get it wrong with this naughty sex position when you are trying to hit on the G-Spot for more erotic stimulation. This sex position brings horniness any time the partners think about sex. This is a hot and sizzling hot position to try out. This sex position is both pleasuring for the man and woman though it will enable the man to hit the woman G-spot easily and in no time. The woman will kneel in front of the man and the man will be behind her and penetrate the woman from behind. Once the man is inside the woman, the woman will then grab the man's ankles as the man will now slowly lift himself to stand supporting the woman with the slightly bent lap. To add more erotic twist the woman should add a lube to her clitoris and squeeze her pelvic muscles along with the thrusts for great session of sex passion.

· Lotus Blossom Position

Lotus sex position is an amazing G-spot stimulating sex position partners can employ to mesmerize one another in the bedroom. This sex position is sure to help give the partners spine tingling orgasm that both deserved. If you are thinking of a sex position you both can relish and will allow great access to G-spot stimulation then you need to try out the Lotus blossom sex position it will surely makes the woman squirts as many times as possible and the man having all the orgasmic thrills from an awesome sex session. This sex position starts with the man sitting down on his butt with his legs crossed while the woman will be fairly close in front of the man almost like the yoga pose and she will sit on the man's crotch facing him, the woman can hold on to the man tightly by wrapping her arms around his back and putting her leg around the man's back too, then she pulls the man more tightly into her vagina and the man hold her firmly too by putting his arm around her. To add more sensation and stimulation the man's hands at the back can be used for a massage and rub the clit while the woman can be grinding and rocking the cock and dry humping. The man will be having a grinding motion until the two partners erupt in an uncontrollable ecstasy. The man can go harder to stimulate the woman more and hit the G-spot stronger. This will aid the breast bouncing more by the woman and this sight alone is erotic for more thrills for the man. The woman can reciprocate the rhythm by throwing her booty back and forth so that both can finally explode in multiple orgasms.

·   Hot Half Headstand

If you are looking for the optimal G-spot stimulating G-spot sex position, then going with the hot half headstand will be the best bet. This is one sex position that both partners can enjoy great stimulations on the genitals and a great way of working through the kinks together. This sex position is very popular with erotic stimulations because it does direct and help partners readjust to a position that they will be able to hit their G-spot easily to get the immense pleasure needed.

This position will have the woman bending in front of the man, the man kneels behind the woman to penetrate from that angle, and the man will fold forward touching the woman. The woman will then grab the man's ankles as she raises her legs to the man side for deep stimulation and easy accessibility of hitting her G-spot. If the partners cannot hold longer at the position, then they can fall back to the missionary position and for more stimulation a rabbit vibrator can be used for ultimate sensual experience.

· Carnal Craving Sex Position

Carnal craving sex position is one sex position that gives partners total control over depth, angle, pace, speed and even the stimulation level during sex session and as such it will help the man get all the thrills that comes with the session while helping gets the woman G-spot well stimulated to the seventh heavens. Both partners will be sure of quenching their lusty desires with this sultry sex position as they explore their bodies and hit all the needed spots to arouse them. The partners begin this position by sitting and facing one another. Then the man grabs the woman waist and under her butt and lift her towards himself and drop her on his laps. The woman will wrap her arms behind the man 's neck and her legs around the man's waist for additional support and the woman will help direct the man's cock into her vagina. In contrast, the man will thrust away at a rhythmic pace. The man can heighten the pleasure by pressing the cock sometimes on the woman's clits.

· Octopus Sex Position

Octopus sex position is an erotic sex position that gives the man the advantage of lasting longer and also giving the woman the opportunity of getting highly stimulated so that the man can hit her G-spot easily. This sex position offers both partner spines tingling orgasm and out of breath ecstasy as they continue to explore one another body and hitting on all the sensual spots to explore in multiple orgasms. With this sex position the man sits on the floor and lean backwards slightly, he can placed his hands behind his back for support then spread his legs a bit to balance himself, then bend his legs slightly afterwards, The woman will stand over the man, with her feet on either side of the man's waist and slowly lower herself on the cock or just squat on your cock, she will direct the cock to her vagina, once the cock is inside her she then sit on your lap and slowly lean backward. She lifts her right leg and leave it at the man's left shoulder while lifting the left leg and keeping it on the man's right shoulders. The man now start thrusting in and out now and intermittently change angle to be able to stimulate the G-spot, The man can use his fingers to rub her clit and press his cock a bit on her clit. The man can make the woman let out all kind of moaning sounds by reaching forward to suck the woman's clit, then penetrate and thrust harder again till both climaxed.

· Coital Alignment Technique {c a t}

Coital alignment technique is an awesome sex position that will be sexually fulfilling for both partners. This sex position enable the man hit directly on the woman's G-spot because this sex position aid change the alignment of the woman's pelvis allowing the man pubic bone to rub against the girl's clitoris now delivering heighten sexual excitement to both partners. This sex position will be great for a little shy and naïve partner as well as beginners that need some easy to maneuver sex positions that are a lot easy to use. CAT can help partners get intimate with themselves as they explore one another bodies. This sex position can be started in the missionary way; the woman will be on her back and the man will be on top of her between her legs. The man now pulls himself up toward the woman's heads that his pelvis is a bit higher up on the girl's body, so instead of the man thrusting in and out, he would rather do more of grinding against the woman's pelvis. For more intense pleasure and to stimulate the G-spot more the man can help the woman part her labia apart so that his body rubs directly against the woman's clitoris or better still keep a pillow under the girl's hips to get more accessible angle. Lastly, the man can use some lube on the girl's clitoris to create a very extra slippery sensation when it touched. With this position the partners are sure of satisfying themselves perfectly.

- ### Devilish Doggy

Devilish doggy is a perfect sex position for hitting on the G-spot; this sex position can be described as the revamp version of the classic cowgirl. It helps both partners discover all the sensual and erotic spots on their body which only brings heavenly pleasure. This sex position will always leave the partner asking for more as the pleasure one another. Devilish doggy is a classic sex position which the woman goes down all four (both on her hands and knees) while the man pleasure and stimulate her from behind. With this position, the rear entry of penetration creates a perfect amount of friction for both partners and of course it helps the man get a deeper penetration to elicit more pleasurable sensation while stimulating and hitting the woman's G-spot. This sex position begins with the woman kneeling and keeping her hands on the floor, the man also kneels behind her upright and penetrate the lady while holding her waist for support. The man can now start thrusting, intermittently the woman will part her legs a little wider so that the man can access her clitoris and can now play with it using the penis. Later the woman can take over too, by the man laying over the edge of the bed and the woman will straddle over the man and stretching her hands towards the man's feet. This will give the man a better view of the woman's body; of course, this sultry view will arouse the man even more. A sex toy can be introduced at this point to help stimulate the woman's G-spot even more too to build up orgasm for both partners before both erupt in a volcanic orgasm.

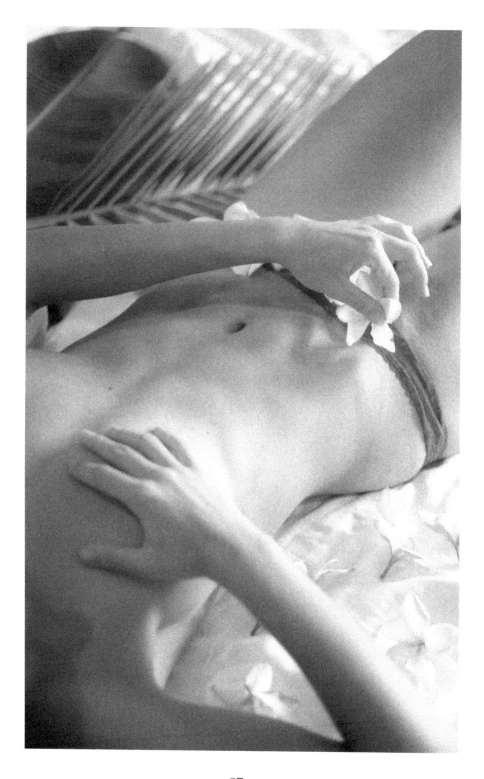

Conclusion

Thank you for making it to the end. You have finally managed to wrap the book and we hope that you have learned a great deal from it. Like we had mentioned at the start of the book, it was not meant to be merely read but it was to be acted upon which we hope you did.

So, re-read the book as many times as needed and you can always choose some of your top favorite experimental positions and please your partner in bed. Everything we have spoken about in the book assumes gargantuan importance and we hope that by reading this book, you must have been able to bring in the much-needed change in your sex life.

Give yourself some time and keep practicing. Being a newbie at sex isn't a really bad thing. In fact, you're exploring and learning a lot of wonderful things about your partner's body as well as your own. You will one day know how to understand your partner's desires and communicate your own – even without words.

So, be willing to do your bit and bring changes for the good. When you are getting a good amount of sex and you are enjoying it, the contentment always shows on your face and this is bound to bring in a rejuvenated sense of joy in you.

So, stay young and wild and feel free to indulge in sex, after all, we all have needs that we need to address. Find your comfort zone and make sure to get out of it once in a while because everyone likes to keep it a little rough and steamy when it comes to sex.

Have a great bedroom game tonight!

Thank you for reading!